The Complete Diabetic Breakfast Cooking Guide

50 fantastic quick and delicious recipes to start the day

Roseann Smith

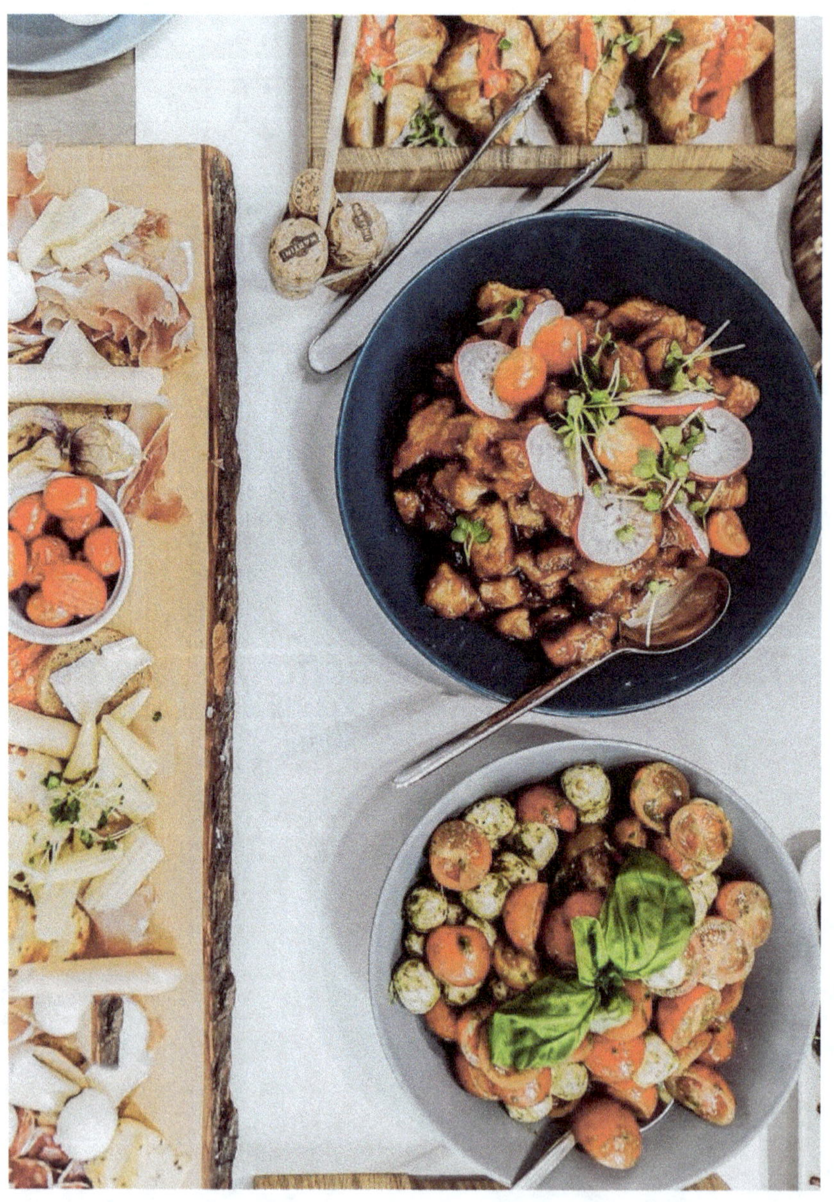

Disclaimer Notice:

Please note the information contained within this document is for educational and entertainment purposes only. All effort has been executed to present accurate, up to date, and reliable, complete information. No warranties of any kind are declared or implied. Readers acknowledge that the author is not engaging in the rendering of legal, financial, medical or professional advice. The content within this book has been derived from various sources. Please consult a licensed professional before attempting any techniques outlined in this book.

By reading this document, the reader agrees that under no circumstances is the author responsible for any losses, direct or indirect, which are incurred as a result of the use of information contained within this document, including, but not limited to, — errors, omissions, or inaccuracies.

Table of Contents

Spiced Overnight Oats

Servings: 6

Cooking Time: None

Ingredients:

- 2 cups old-fashioned oats
- 1 cup fat-free milk
- 1 tablespoon vanilla extract
- 1 teaspoon liquid stevia extract
- 1 teaspoon ground cinnamon
- ¼ teaspoon ground nutmeg
- ½ cup toasted walnuts, chopped

Directions:

1. Stir together the oats, milk, vanilla extract, liquid stevia extract, cinnamon, and nutmeg in a large bowl.
2. Cover and chill overnight until thick.
3. Stir in the yogurt just before serving and spoon into cups.

4. Top with chopped walnuts and fresh fruit to serve.

Nutrition Info: Calories 140, Total Fat 7.1g, Saturated Fat 0.5g, Total Carbs 12.7g, Net Carbs 10.4g, Protein 5.6g, Sugar 2.6g, Fiber 2.3g, Sodium 23mg

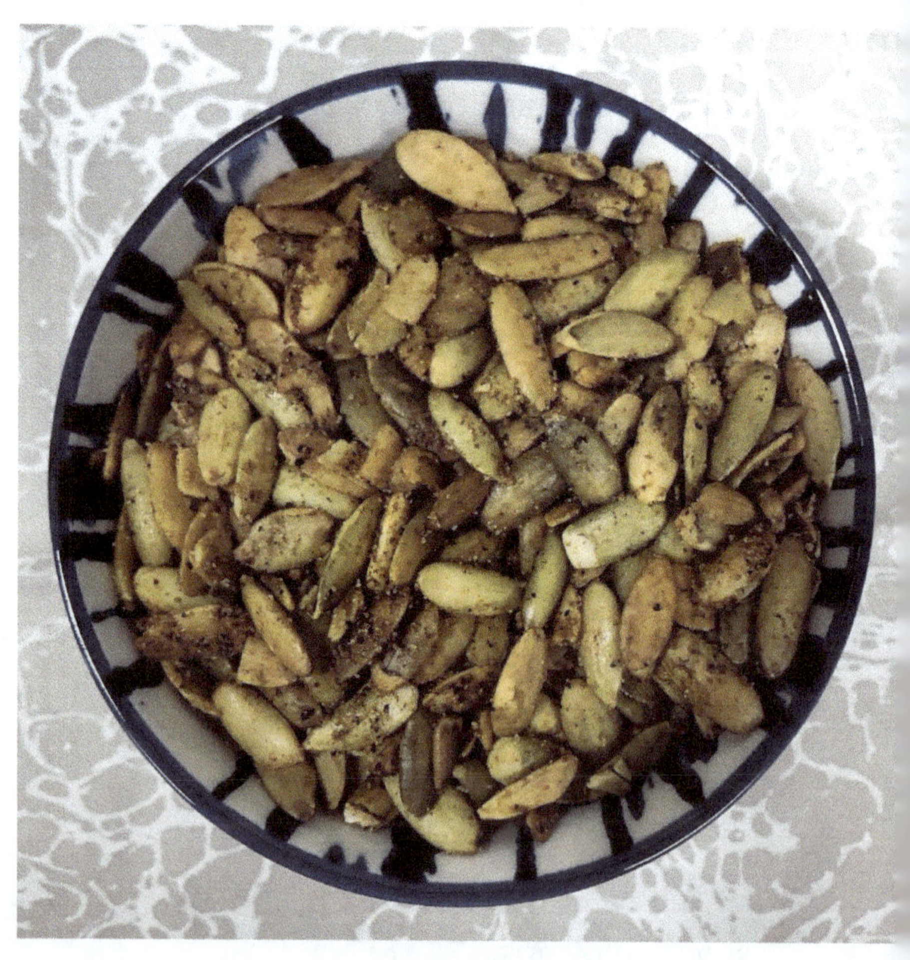

Almond & Berry Smoothie

Servings: 1

Cooking Time: 0 Minute

Ingredients:

- ⅔ cup frozen raspberries
- ½ cup frozen banana, sliced
- ½ cup almond milk (unsweetened)
- 3 tablespoons almonds, sliced
- ¼ teaspoon ground cinnamon
- ⅛ teaspoon vanilla extract
- ¼ cup blueberries
- 1 tablespoon coconut flakes (unsweetened)

Directions:

1. Put the Ingredients in a blender except coconut flakes. Pulse until smooth.
2. Top with the coconut flakes before serving.

Nutrition Info: Calories 360 Total Fat 19 g Saturated Fat 3 g Cholesterol 0 mg Sodium 89 mg Total Carbohydrate 46 g Dietary Fiber 14 g Total Sugars 21 g Protein 9 g Potassium 736 mg

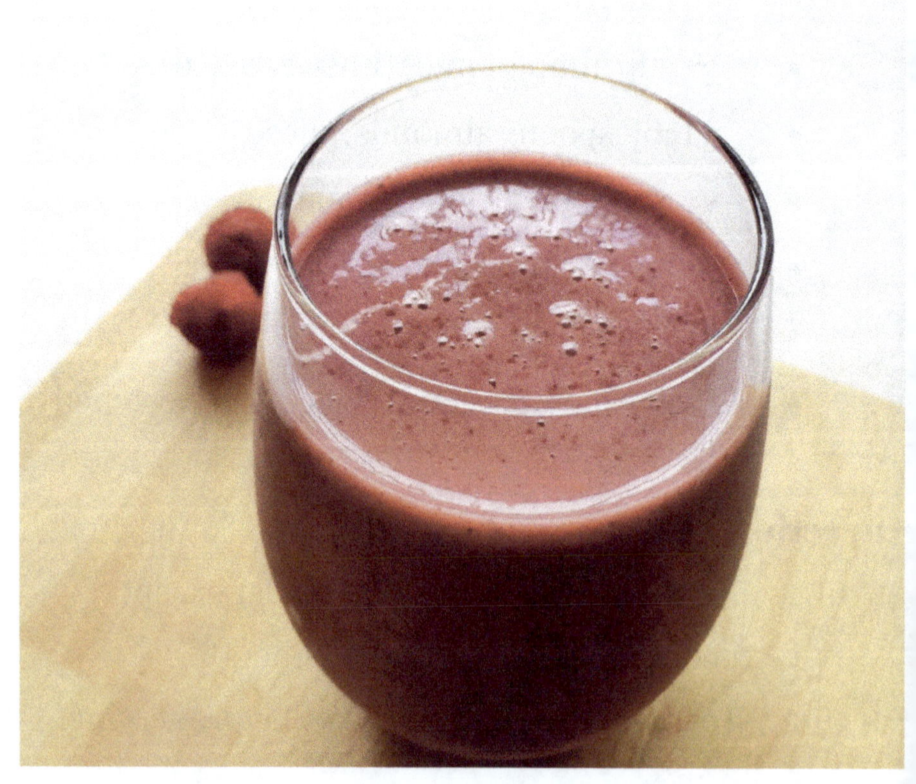

Keto Low Carb Crepe

Servings: 2

Cooking Time: 4 Minutes

Ingredients:

- 2 eggs
- 1 egg white
- 1 tbsp unsalted butter
- 1 1/3 tbsp cream cheese
- 2/3 tbsp psyllium husk

Directions:

1. preparation the batter and for this, put all the ingredients in a bowl, except for butter, and then whisk by using a stick blender until smooth and very liquid.
2. Bring out a skillet pan, put it over medium heat, add ½ tbsp butter and when it melts,

pour in half of the batter, spread evenly, and
cook until the top has firmed.

3. Carefully flip the crepe, then continue
cooking for 2 minutes until cooked and then
move it to a plate.

4. Add remaining butter and when it melts,
cook another crepe in the same manner and
then serve.

Nutrition Info: 118 Cal 9.4 g Fats 6.5 g Protein 1 g
Net Carb 0.9 g Fiber

Cinnamon Oat Pancakes

Servings: 6

Cooking Time: 15 Minutes

Ingredients:

- 1 cup old-fashioned oats
- 1 cup whole-wheat flour
- 2 teaspoons baking powder
- 1 teaspoon salt
- 1 ½ cups fat-free milk
- ¼ cup canola oil
- 2 large eggs, whisked
- 1 teaspoon lemon juice
- ½ to 1 teaspoon liquid stevia extract

Directions:

1. Combine the oats, flour, baking powder, and salt in a medium mixing bowl.
2. In a separate bowl, stir together the milk, canola oil, eggs, lemon juice, and stevia extract.
3. Stir the wet ingredients into the dry until just combined.
4. Heat a large skillet or griddle to medium-high heat and grease with cooking spray.
5. Spoon the batter in ¼ cups into the skillet and cook until bubbles form on the surface.
6. Flip the pancakes and cook to brown on the other side.
7. Slide onto a plate and repeat with the remaining batter.
8. Store the extra pancakes in an airtight container and reheat in the microwave or oven.

Nutrition Info: Calories 230, Total Fat 11.4g, Saturated Fat 1.3g, Total Carbs 24.3g, Net Carbs 23g, Protein 7.1g, Sugar 3.3g, Fiber 1.3g, Sodium 446mg

Yogurt And Kale Smoothie

Servings: 1

Ingredients:

- 1 cup whole milk yogurt
- 1 cup baby kale greens
- 1 pack stevia
- 1 tablespoon MCT oil
- 1 tablespoon sunflower seeds
- 1 cup of water

Directions:

1. Add listed ingredients to the blender
2. Blend until you have a smooth and creamy texture
3. Serve chilled and enjoy!

Nutrition Info: Calories: 329; Fat: 26g; Carbohydrates: 15g; Protein: 11g

Healthy Carrot Muffins

Servings: 8

Cooking Time: 40 Minutes

Ingredients:

- Dry ingredients
- Tapioca starch – ¼ cup
- Baking soda – 1 teaspoon
- Cinnamon – 1 tablespoon
- Cloves – ¼ teaspoon
- Wet ingredients
- Vanilla extract – 1 teaspoon
- Water – 11/2 cups
- Carrots (shredded) – 11/2 cups
- Almond flour – 1¾ cups
- Granulated sweetener of choice – 1/2 cup
- Baking powder – 1 teaspoon
- Nutmeg – 1 teaspoon
- Salt – 1 teaspoon

- Coconut oil – 1/3 cup
- Flax meal – 4 tablespoons
- Banana (mashed) – 1 medium

Directions:

1. Begin by heating the oven to 350F.
2. Get a muffin tray and position paper cups in all the moulds. Arrange aside.
3. Get a small glass bowl and put half a cup of water and flax meal. Allow this rest for about 5 minutes. Your flax egg is prepared.
4. Get a large mixing bowl and put in the almond flour, tapioca starch, granulated sugar, baking soda, baking powder, cinnamon, nutmeg, cloves, and salt. Mix well to combine.
5. Conform a well in the middle of the flour mixture and stream in the coconut oil, vanilla extract, and flax egg. Mix well to conform a mushy dough.
6. Then put in the chopped carrots and mashed banana. Mix until well-combined.

7. Make use of a spoon to scoop out an equal amount of mixture into 8 muffin cups.

8. Position the muffin tray in the oven and allow it to bake for about 40 minutes.

9. Extract the tray from the microwave and allow the muffins to stand for about 10 minutes.

10. Extract the muffin cups from the tray and allow them to chill until they reach room degree of hotness and coldness.

11. Serve and enjoy!

Nutrition Info: Calories: 189 calories per serving; Fat 13.9 g; Protein 3.8 g; Carbs 17.3 g

Breakfast Smoothie Bowl With Fresh Berries

Servings: 2

Cooking Time: 5 Minutes

Ingredients:

- Almond milk (unsweetened) – 1/2 cup
- Psyllium husk powder – 1/2 teaspoon
- Strawberries (chopped) – 2 ounces
- Coconut oil – 1 tablespoon
- Crushed ice – 3 cups
- Liquid stevia – 5 to 10 drops
- Pea protein powder – 1/3 cup

Directions:

1. Begin by taking a blender and adding in the mashed ice cubes. Allow them to rest for about 30 seconds.

2. Then put in the almond milk, shredded strawberries, pea protein powder, psyllium

husk powder, coconut oil, and liquid stevia.
Blend well until it turns into a smooth and
creamy puree.

3. Vacant the prepared smoothie into 2 glasses.
4. Cover with coconut flakes and pure and neat
    strawberries.

Nutrition Info: Calories: 166 calories per serving; Fat
– 9.2 g; Carbs – 4.1 g; Protein – 17.6 g

Keto Creamy Bacon Dish

Servings: 2

Cooking Time: 5 Minutes

Ingredients:

- ½ tsp dried basil
- ½ tsp minced garlic
- ½ tsp tomato paste
- 2 oz unsalted butter, softened
- 3 slices of bacon, chopped

Directions:

1. Bring out a skillet pan, put it over medium heat, add 1 tbsp butter and when it starts to melts, add chopped bacon and cook for 5 minutes.
2. Then remove the pan from heat, add remaining butter, along with basil and tomato paste, season with salt and black pepper and stir until well mixed.

3.   Move bacon butter into an airtight container, cover with the lid, and refrigerate for 1 hour until solid.

Nutrition Info: 150 Cal 16 g Fats 1 g Protein 0.5 g Net Carb 1 g Fiber

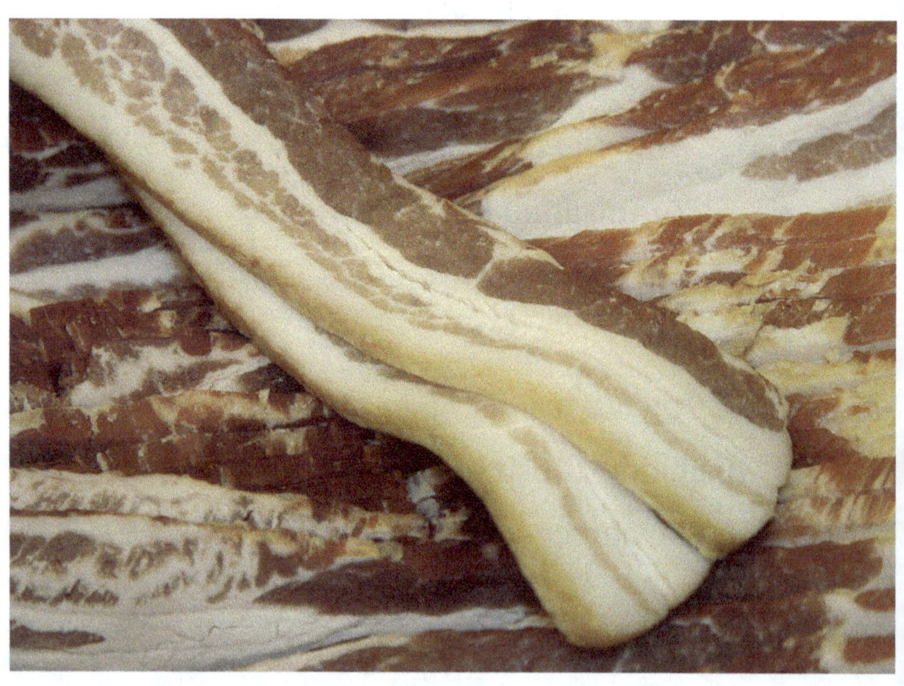

Egg "dough" In A Pan

Servings: 2

Cooking Time: 4 Minutes

Ingredients:

- ¼ tsp salt
- ½ of medium red bell pepper, chopped
- 1/8 tsp ground black pepper
- 2 eggs
- 2 tbsp chopped chives

Directions:

1. Turn on the oven, then set it to 350 degrees F and let it preheat.
2. In the meantime, crack eggs in a bowl, add remaining ingredients and whisk until combined.
3. Bring out a small heatproof dish, pour in egg mixture, and bake for 5 to 8 minutes until set.

4.   When done, cut it into two squares and then serve.

Nutrition Info: 87 Cal 5.4 g Fats 7.2 g Protein 1.7 g Net Carb 0.7 g Fiber

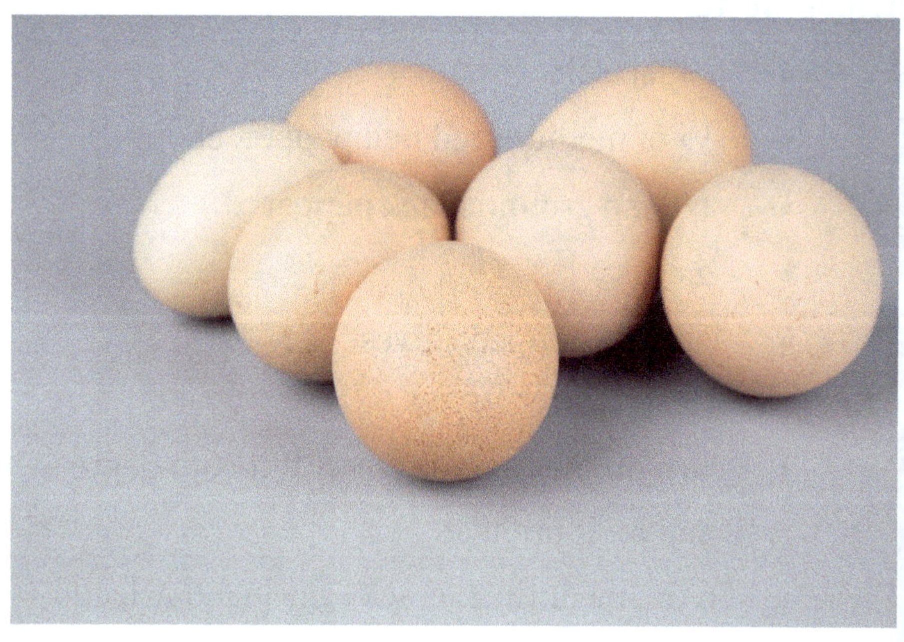

Greek Chicken Breast

Servings: 4

Cooking Time: 25 Minutes

Ingredients:

- 4 chicken breast halves, skinless and boneless
- 1 cup extra virgin olive oil
- 1 lemon, juiced
- 2 teaspoons garlic, crushed
- 1 and 1/2 teaspoons black pepper
- 1/3 teaspoon paprika

Directions:

1. Cut 3 slits in the chicken breast
2. Take a small bowl and whisk in olive oil, salt, lemon juice, garlic, paprika, pepper and whisk for 30 seconds
3. Place chicken in a large bowl and pour marinade

4. Rub the marinade all over using your hand

5. Refrigerate overnight

6. Pre-heat grill to medium heat and oil the grate

7. Cook chicken in the grill until center is no longer pink

8. Serve and enjoy!

Nutrition Info: Calories: 644; Fat: 57g; Carbohydrates: 2g; Protein: 27g

Eggs Florentine

Servings: 2

Cooking Time: 10 Minutes

Ingredients:

- 1 cup washed, fresh spinach leaves
- 2 tbsp freshly grated parmesan cheese
- Sea salt and pepper
- 1 tbsp white vinegar
- 2 eggs

Directions:

1. Cook the spinach the microwave or steam until wilted.
2. Sprinkle with parmesan cheese and seasoning.
3. Slice into bite-size pieces
4. Simmer a pan of water and add the vinegar. Stir quickly with a spoon.

5.   Break an egg into the center. Turn off the heat and cover until set.

6.   Repeat with the second egg.

7.   Place the eggs on top of the spinach and serve.

Nutrition Info: 180 cal.10g fat 7g protein 5g carbs.

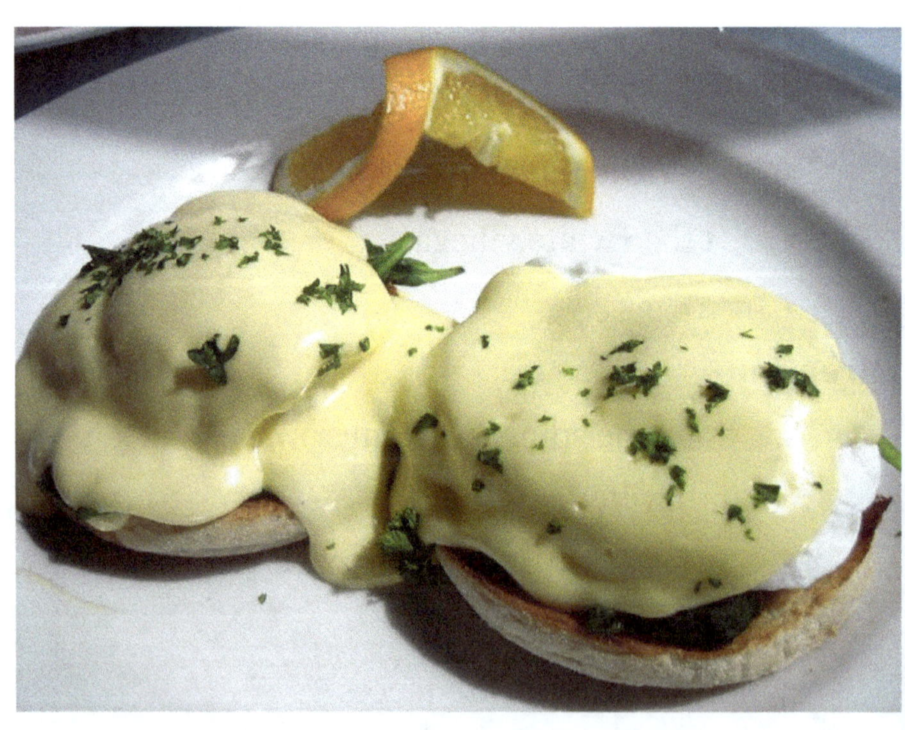

Healthy Baked Eggs

Servings: 6

Cooking Time: 1 Hour

Ingredients:

- Olive oil – 1 tablespoon
- Garlic – 2 cloves
- Eggs – 8 large
- Sea salt – 1/2 teaspoon
- Shredded mozzarella cheese (medium-fat) – 3 cups
- Olive oil spray
- Onion (chopped) – 1 medium
- Spinach leaves – 8 ounces
- Half-and-half – 1 cup
- Black pepper – 1 teaspoon
- Feta cheese – 1/2 cup

Directions:

1. Begin by heating the oven to 375F.
2. Get a glass baking dish and grease it with olive oil spray. Arrange aside.
3. Now take a nonstick pan and pour in the olive oil. Position the pan on allows heat and allows it heat.
4. Immediately you are done, toss in the garlic, spinach, and onion. Prepare for about 5 minutes. Arrange aside.
5. You can now Get a large mixing bowl and add in the half, eggs, pepper, and salt. Whisk thoroughly to combine.
6. Put in the feta cheese and chopped mozzarella cheese (reserve 1/2 cup of mozzarella cheese for later).
7. Put the egg mixture and prepared spinach to the prepared glass baking dish. Blend well to combine. Drizzle the reserved cheese over the top.

8. Bake the egg mix for about 45 minutes.

9. Extract the baking dish from the oven and allow it to stand for 10 minutes.

10. Dice and serve!

Nutrition Info: Calories: 323 calories per serving; Fat 22.3 g; Protein 22.6 g; Carbs 7.9 g

Quick Low-carb Oatmeal

Servings: 2

Cooking Time: 15 Minutes

Ingredients:

- Almond flour – 1/2 cup
- Flax meal – 2 tablespoons
- Cinnamon (ground) – 1 teaspoon
- Almond milk (unsweetened) – 11/2 cups
- Salt – as per taste
- Chia seeds – 2 tablespoons
- Liquid stevia – 10 – 15 drops
- Vanilla extract – 1 teaspoon

Directions:

1. Begin by taking a large mixing bowl and adding in the coconut flour, almond flour, ground cinnamon, flax seed powder, and chia seeds. Mix properly to combine.

2. Position a stockpot on a low heat and add in the dry ingredients. Also add in the liquid stevia, vanilla extract, and almond milk. Mix well to combine.

3. Prepare the flour and almond milk for about 4 minutes. Add salt if needed.

4. Move the oatmeal to a serving bowl and top with nuts, seeds, and pure and neat berries.

Nutrition Info: Calories: calories per serving; Protein – 11.7 g; Fat – 24.3 g; Carbs – 16.7 g

Balsamic Chicken

Servings: 6

Cooking Time: 25 Minutes

Ingredients:

- 6 chicken breast halves, skinless and boneless
- 1 teaspoon garlic salt
- Ground black pepper
- 2 tablespoons olive oil
- 1 onion, thinly sliced
- 14 and 1/2 ounces tomatoes, diced
- 1/2 cup balsamic vinegar
- 1 teaspoon dried basil
- 1 teaspoon dried oregano
- 1 teaspoon dried rosemary
- 1/2 teaspoon dried thyme

Directions:

1. Season both sides of your chicken breasts thoroughly with pepper and garlic salt
2. Take a skillet and place it over medium heat
3. Add some oil and cook your seasoned chicken for 3-4 minutes per side until the breasts are nicely browned
4. Add some onion and cook for another 3-4 minutes until the onions are browned
5. Pour the diced up tomatoes and balsamic vinegar over your chicken and season with some rosemary, basil, thyme, and rosemary
6. Simmer the chicken for about 15 minutes until they are no longer pink
7. Take an instant-read thermometer and check if the internal temperature gives a reading of 165 degrees Fahrenheit
8. If yes, then you are good to go!

Nutrition Info: Calories: 196; Fat: 7g; Carbohydrates: 7g; Protein: 23g

Vegetable Noodles Stir-fry

Servings: 4

Cooking Time: 40 Minutes

Ingredients:

- White sweet potato – 1 pound
- Zucchini – 8 ounces
- Garlic cloves (finely chopped) – 2 large
- Vegetable broth – 2 tablespoons
- Salt – as per taste
- Carrots – 8 ounces
- Shallot (finely chopped) – 1
- Red chili (finely chopped) – 1
- Olive oil – 1 tablespoon
- Pepper – as per taste

Directions:

1. Begin by scrapping the carrots and sweet potato. Make Use a spiralizer to make noodles out of the sweet potato and carrots.

2. Rinse the zucchini thoroughly and spiralize it as well.

3. Get a large skillet and position it on a high flame. Stream in the vegetable broth and allow it to come to a boil.

4. Toss in the spiralized sweet potato and carrots. Then put in the chili, garlic, and shallots. Stir everything using tongs and cook for some minutes.

5. Transfer the vegetable noodles into a serving platter and generously spice with pepper and salt.

6. Finalize by sprinkling olive oil over the noodles. Serve while hot!

Nutrition Info: Calories: 169 calories per serving; Fat 3.7 g; Protein 3.6 g; Carbs – 31.2 g

Cucumber & Yogurt

Servings: 1

Cooking Time: 0 Minute

Ingredients:

- 1 cup low-fat yogurt
- ½ cup cucumber, diced
- ¼ teaspoon lemon zest
- ¼ teaspoon lemon juice
- ¼ teaspoon fresh mint, chopped
- Salt to taste

Directions:

1. Mix all the Ingredients in a jar.
2. Refrigerate and serve.

Nutrition Info: Calories 164 Total Fat 4 g Saturated Fat 2 g Cholesterol 15 mg Sodium 318 mg Total Carbohydrate 19 g Dietary Fiber 1 g Total Sugars 18 g Protein 13 g Potassium 683 mg

Eggs Baked In Peppers

Servings: 4

Cooking Time: 25 Minutes

Ingredients:

- 4 medium bell peppers, assorted
- 1 cup shredded low-fat cheddar cheese
- 8 large eggs
- Salt and pepper
- Fresh chopped parsley, to serve

Directions:

1. Preheat the oven to 400°F and slice the peppers in half.
2. Remove the seeds and pith from each pepper and place them cut-side up in a baking dish large enough to fit them all.
3. Divide the shredded cheese among the pepper halves and crack an egg into each.

4.   Season with salt and pepper then bake for 20 to 25 minutes until done to your liking.

5.   Garnish with fresh chopped parsley to serve.

Nutrition Info: Calories 260, Total Fat 16.3g, Saturated Fat 6.6g, Total Carbs 10.9g, Net Carbs 9.3g, Protein 20.8g, Sugar 6.8g, Fiber 1.6g, Sodium 374mg

Easy Egg Scramble

Servings: 1

Cooking Time: 10 Minutes

Ingredients:

- 2 large eggs
- 1 tablespoon fat-free milk
- Salt and pepper
- ¼ cup diced green pepper
- 2 tablespoons diced onion
- ¼ cup diced tomatoes

Directions:

1. Whisk together the eggs, milk, salt, and pepper in a small bowl.
2. Heat a medium skillet over medium-high heat and grease with cooking spray.
3. Add the green pepper and onion then cook for 2 to 3 minutes.

4. Spoon the veggies into a bowl then reheat the skillet.

5. Pour in the egg mixture and cook until the eggs start to thicken.

6. Spoon in the cooked veggies and diced tomatoes.

7. Stir the mixture and cook until the egg is set and scrambled. Serve hot.

Nutrition Info: Calories 170, Total Fat 10.1g, Saturated Fat 3.1g, Total Carbs 6.3g, Net Carbs 4.9g, Protein 13.9g, Sugar 4.1g, Fiber 1.4g, Sodium 152mg

Bacon And Chicken Garlic Wrap

Servings: 4

Cooking Time: 10 Minutes

Ingredients:

- 1 chicken fillet, cut into small cubes
- 8-9 thin slices bacon, cut to fit cubes
- 6 garlic cloves, minced

Directions:

1. Preheat your oven to 400 degrees F
2. Line a baking tray with aluminum foil
3. Add minced garlic to a bowl and rub each chicken piece with it
4. Wrap bacon piece around each garlic chicken bite
5. Secure with toothpick
6. Transfer bites to the baking sheet, keeping a little bit of space between them
7. Bake for about 15-20 minutes until crispy

8. Serve and enjoy!

Nutrition Info: Calories: 260; Fat: 19g; Carbohydrates: 5g; Protein: 22g

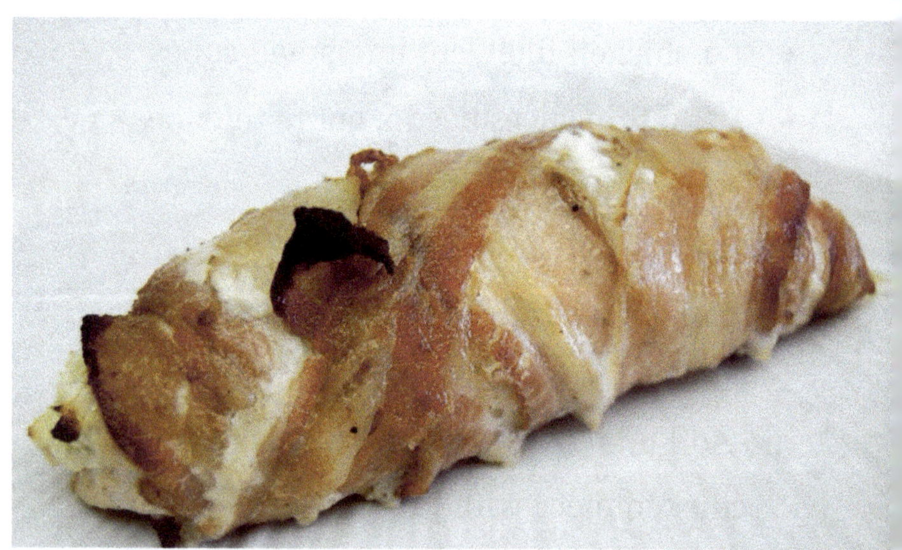

Strawberry Puff Pancake

Servings: 4

Cooking Time: 20 Minutes

Ingredients:

- 3 eggs, large
- 1/8 teaspoon cinnamon, ground
- 1 cup strawberry, sliced
- 3/4 cup milk, fat-free
- What you will need from the store cupboard:
- 1 teaspoon vanilla extract
- ¾ cup of all-purpose flour
- 2 tablespoons of butter
- 1 tablespoon cornstarch
- ½ cup of water
- 1/8 teaspoon salt

Directions:

1. Keep the butter in a pie plate and keep in an oven for 4 to 5 minutes.
2. In the meantime, whisk the vanilla, milk, and eggs in a bowl.
3. Take another bowl and bring together the cinnamon, salt, and flour in it.
4. Whisk this into the egg mix until it blends well. Pour this into the plate.
5. Bake for 15 minutes. The sides should be golden brown and crisp.
6. Add the cornstarch in your saucepan. Stir the water in until it turns smooth.
7. Now add the strawberries. Cook while stirring till it thickens.
8. Mash the strawberries coarsely and serve with the pancake.

Nutrition Info: Calories 277, Carbohydrates 38g, Fiber 2g, Cholesterol 175mg, Total Fat 10g, Protein 9g, Sodium 187mg

Egg Porridge

Servings: 1

Cooking Time: 10 Minutes

Ingredients:

- 2 organic free-range eggs
- 1/3 cup organic heavy cream without food additives
- 2 packages of your preferred sweetener
- 2 tbsp grass-fed butter ground organic cinnamon to taste

Directions:

1. In a bowl add the eggs, cream and sweetener, and mix together.
2. Melt the butter in a saucepan over a medium heat. Lower the heat once the butter is melted.
3. Combine together with the egg and cream mixture.

4.   While Cooking, mix until it thickens and curdles.

5.   When you see the first signs of curdling, remove the saucepan immediately from the heat.

6.   Pour the porridge into a bowl. Sprinkle cinnamon on top and serve immediately.

Nutrition Info: 604 cal 45g fat 8g protein 2.8g carbs.

Chipotle Lettuce Chicken

Servings: 6

Cooking Time: 25 Minutes

Ingredients:

- 1 pound chicken breast, cut into strips
- Splash of olive oil
- 1 red onion, finely sliced
- 14 ounces tomatoes
- 1 teaspoon chipotle, chopped
- 1/2 teaspoon cumin
- Pinch of sugar
- Lettuce as needed
- Fresh coriander leaves
- Jalapeno chilies, sliced
- Fresh tomato slices for garnish
- Lime wedges

Directions:

1. Take a non-stick frying pan and place it over medium heat
2. Add oil and heat it up
3. Add chicken and cook until brown
4. Keep the chicken on the side
5. Add tomatoes, sugar, chipotle, cumin to the same pan and simmer for 25 minutes until you have a nice sauce
6. Add chicken into the sauce and cook for 5 minutes
7. Transfer the mix to another place
8. Use lettuce wraps to take a portion of the mixture and serve with a squeeze of lemon
9. Enjoy!

Nutrition Info: Calories: 332; Fat: 15g; Carbohydrates: 13g; Protein: 34g

Breakfast Parfait

Servings: 2

Cooking Time: 0 Minute

Ingredients:

- 4 oz. unsweetened applesauce
- 6 oz. non-fat and sugar-free vanilla yogurt
- ¼ teaspoon pumpkin pie spice
- ¼ teaspoon honey
- 1 cup low-fat granola

Directions:

1. Mix the Ingredients except the granola in a bowl.
2. Layer the mixture with the granola in a cup.
3. Refrigerate before serving.

Nutrition Info: Calories 287 Total Fat 3 g Saturated Fat 1 g Cholesterol 28 mg Sodium 186 mg Total Carbohydrate 57 g Dietary Fiber 4 g Total Sugars2 g Protein 8 g Potassium 4

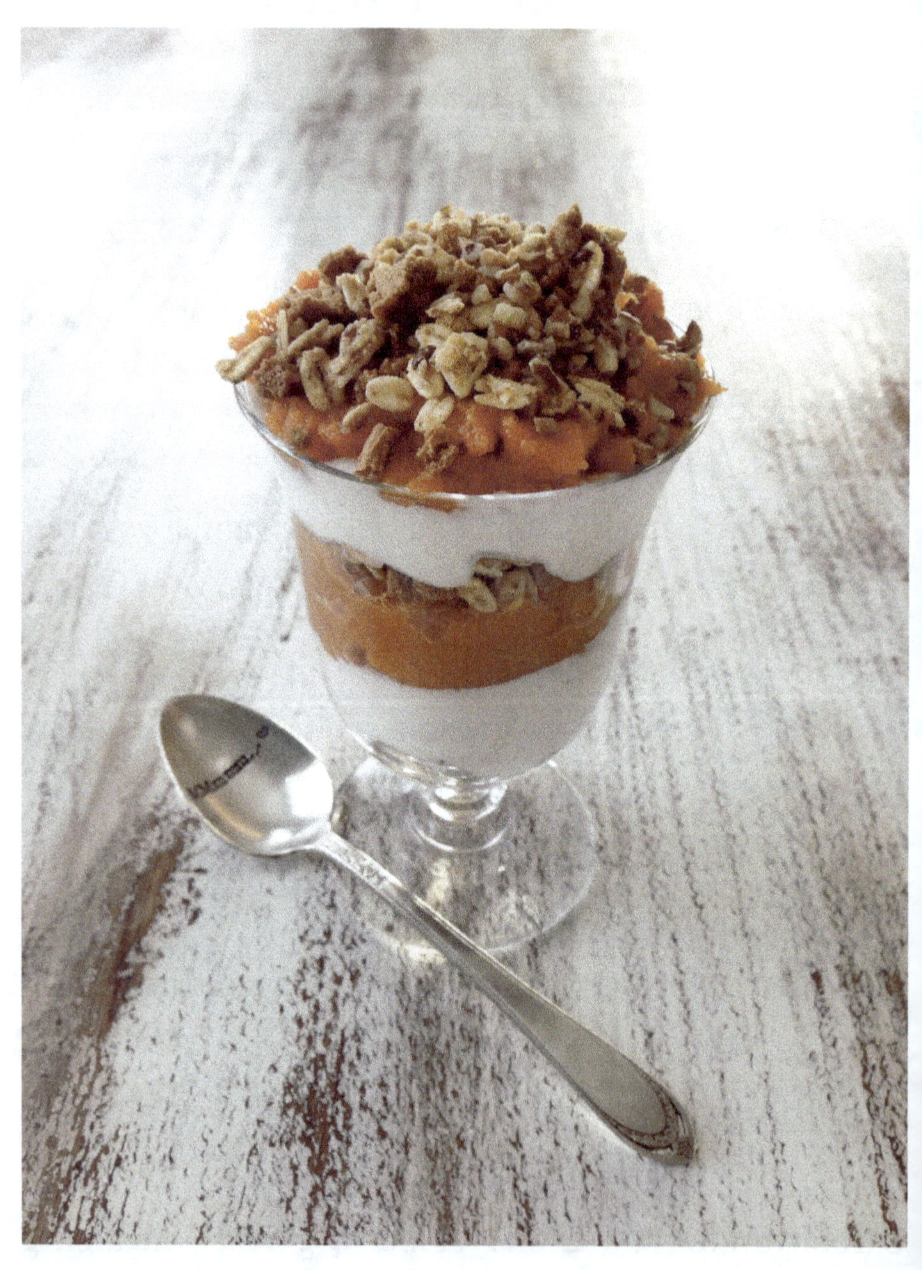

Oatmeal Blueberry Pancakes

Servings: 4

Cooking Time: 40 Minutes

Ingredients:

- ½ cup rolled oats
- ½ cup unsweetened almond milk
- ¼ cup unsweetened applesauce
- ¼ cup unsweetened vegan protein powder
- ½ tablespoon flax meal
- 1 teaspoon baking powder
- ½ teaspoon vanilla extract
- ¼ teaspoon baking soda
- ¼ teaspoon ground cinnamon
- 1/8 teaspoon salt
- ½ cup fresh blueberries

Directions:

1. Place all ingredients (except for blueberries) in a food processor and pulse until smooth.
2. Transfer the mixture into a bowl and set aside for 5 minutes.
3. Gently, fold in blueberries.
4. Place a lightly greased medium skillet over medium heat until heated.
5. Place desired amount of the mixture and cook for about 3–5 minutes per side.
6. Repeat with the remaining mixture.
7. Serve warm.

Nutrition Info: Calories 105 Total Fat 1.8 g Saturated Fat 0.2 g Cholesterol 0 mg Sodium 204 mg Total Carbs 15.4 g Fiber 2.2 g Sugar 5.2 g Protein 8 g

Bulgur Porridge

Servings: 2

Cooking Time: 15 Minutes

Ingredients:

- 2/3 cup unsweetened soy milk
- 1/3 cup bulgur, rinsed
- Pinch of salt
- 1 ripe banana, peeled and mashed
- 2 kiwis, peeled and sliced

Directions:

1. In a pan, add the soy milk, bulgur, and salt over medium-high heat and bring to a boil.
2. Adjust the heat to low and simmer for about 10 minutes.
3. Remove the pan of bulgur from heat and immediately, stir in the mashed banana.
4. Serve warm with the topping of kiwi slices.

Nutrition Info: Calories 223 Total Fat 2.3 g
Saturated Fat 0.3 g Cholesterol 0 mg Sodium 126 mg
Total Carbs 47.5 g Fiber 8.6 g Sugar 17.4 g Protein 7.1 g

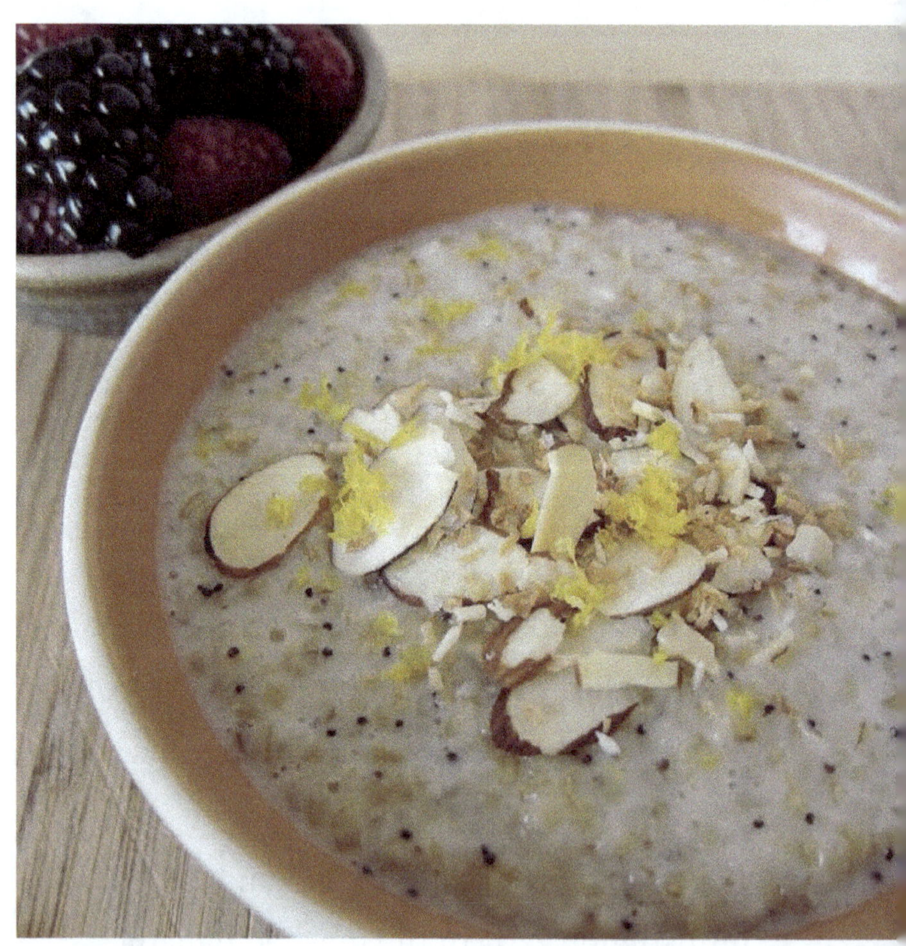

Turkey-broccoli Brunch Casserole

Servings: 6

Cooking Time: 20 Minutes

Ingredients:

- 2-1/2 cups turkey breast, cubed and cooked
- 16 oz. broccoli, chopped and drained
- 1-1/2 cups of milk, fat-free
- 1 cup cheddar cheese, low-fat, shredded
- 10 oz. cream of chicken soup. low sodium and low fat
- What you will need from the store cupboard:
- 8 oz. egg substitute
- ¼ teaspoon of poultry seasoning
- ¼ cup of sour cream, low fat
- ½ teaspoon pepper
- 1/8 teaspoon salt
- 2 cups of seasoned stuffing cubes

- • Cooking spray

Directions:

1. Bring together the egg substitute, soup, milk, pepper, sour cream, salt, and poultry seasoning in a big bowl.
2. Now stir in the broccoli, turkey, ¾ cup of cheese and stuffing cubes.
3. Transfer to a baking dish. Apply cooking spray.
4. Bake for 10 minutes. Sprinkle the remaining cheese.
5. Bake for another 5 minutes.
6. Keep it aside for 5 minutes. Serve.

Nutrition Info: Calories 303, Carbohydrates 26g, Fiber 3g, Sugar 0.8g, Cholesterol 72mg, Total Fat 7g, Protein 33g

Cheesy Low-carb Omelet

Servings: 5

Cooking Time: 5 Minutes

Ingredients:

- 2 whole eggs
- 1 tablespoon water
- 1 tablespoon butter
- 3 thin slices salami
- 5 fresh basil leaves
- 5 thin slices, fresh ripe tomatoes
- 2 ounces fresh mozzarella cheese
- Salt and pepper as needed

Directions:

1. Take a small bowl and whisk in eggs and water
2. Take a non-stick Sauté pan and place it over medium heat, add butter and let it melt
3. Pour egg mixture and cook for 30 seconds

4. Spread salami slices on half of egg mix and top with cheese, tomatoes, basil slices

5. Season with salt and pepper according to your taste

6. Cook for 2 minutes and fold the egg with the empty half

7. Cover and cook on LOW for 1 minute

8. Serve and enjoy!

Nutrition Info: Calories: 451; Fat: 36g; Carbohydrates: 3g; Protein:33g

Apple & Cinnamon Pancake

Servings: 4

Cooking Time: 10 Minutes

Ingredients:

- ¼ teaspoon ground cinnamon
- 1 ¾ cups Better Baking Mix
- 1 tablespoon oil
- 1 cup water
- 2 egg whites
- ½ cup sugar-free applesauce
- Cooking spray
- 1 cup plain yogurt
- Sugar substitute

Directions:

1. Blend the cinnamon and the baking mix in a bowl.
2. Create a hole in the middle and add the oil, water, egg and applesauce.

3. Mix well.

4. Spray your pan with oil.

5. Place it on medium heat.

6. Pour ¼ cup of the batter.

7. Flip the pancake and cook until golden.

8. Serve with yogurt and sugar substitute.

Nutrition Info: Calories 231 Total Fat 6 g Saturated Fat 1 g Cholesterol 54 mg Sodium 545 mg Total Carbohydrate 37 g Dietary Fiber 4 g Total Sugars 1 g Protein 8 g Potassium 750 mg

Guacamole Turkey Burgers

Servings: 3

Cooking Time: 15 Minutes

Ingredients:

- 12 oz. turkey, ground

- 1-1/2 avocados

- 2 teaspoons of juice from a lime

- ½ teaspoon cumin

- 1 red chili, chopped

- What you will need from the store cupboard:

- ½ teaspoon garlic powder

- ½ teaspoon onion powder

- 3 teaspoons of olive oil

- ½ teaspoon salt

Directions:

1. Mix the turkey with the cumin, chili, salt, garlic powder, and onion powder in a medium-sized bowl.
2. Create 3 patties
3. Pour 3 teaspoons olive oil in a skillet and heat over medium heat.
4. Now cook your patties. Make sure that both sides are brown.
5. Make the guacamole in the meantime.
6. Mash together the garlic powder, juice from lime and avocados in a bowl.
7. Add salt for seasoning.
8. Serve the burgers with guacamole on the patties.

Nutrition Info: Calories 316, Carbohydrates 9g, Fiber 8g, Sugar 0g, Cholesterol 80mg, Total Fat 21g, Protein 24g

Ham And Goat Cheese Omelet

Servings: 1

Cooking Time: 10 Minutes

Ingredients:

- 1 slice of ham, chopped
- 4 egg whites
- 2 teaspoons of water
- 2 tablespoons onion, chopped
- 1 tablespoon parsley, minced
- What you will need from the store cupboard:
- 2 tablespoons green pepper, chopped
- 1/8 teaspoon pepper
- 2 tablespoons goat cheese, crumbled
- Cooking spray

Directions:

1. Whisk together the water, pepper and egg whites in a bowl till everything blends well.
2. Stir in the green pepper, ham, and onion.
3. Now heat your skillet over medium heat after applying the cooking spray.
4. Pour in the egg white mix towards the edge.
5. As it sets, push the cooked parts to the center. Allow the uncooked portions to flow underneath.
6. Sprinkle the goat cheese to one side when there is no liquid egg.
7. Now fold your omelet into half.
8. Sprinkle the parsley.

Nutrition Info: Calories 143, Carbohydrates 5g, Fiber 1g, Sugar 0.3g, Cholesterol 27mg, Total Fat 4g, Protein 21g

Strawberry & Spinach Smoothie

Servings: 2

Cooking Time: 15 Minutes

Ingredients:

- 1½ cups fresh strawberries, hulled and sliced
- 2 cups fresh baby spinach
- ½ cup fat-free plain Greek yogurt
- 1 cup unsweetened almond milk
- ¼ cup ice cubes

Directions:

1. In a high-speed blender, add all the ingredients and pulse until smooth.
2. Pour into serving glasses and serve immediately.

Nutrition Info: Calories 96 Total Fat 2.3 g Saturated Fat 0.2 g Cholesterol 1 mg Total Carbs 12.3 g Sugar 7.7 g Fiber 3.9 g Sodium 144 mg Potassium 428 mg Protein 8.1 g

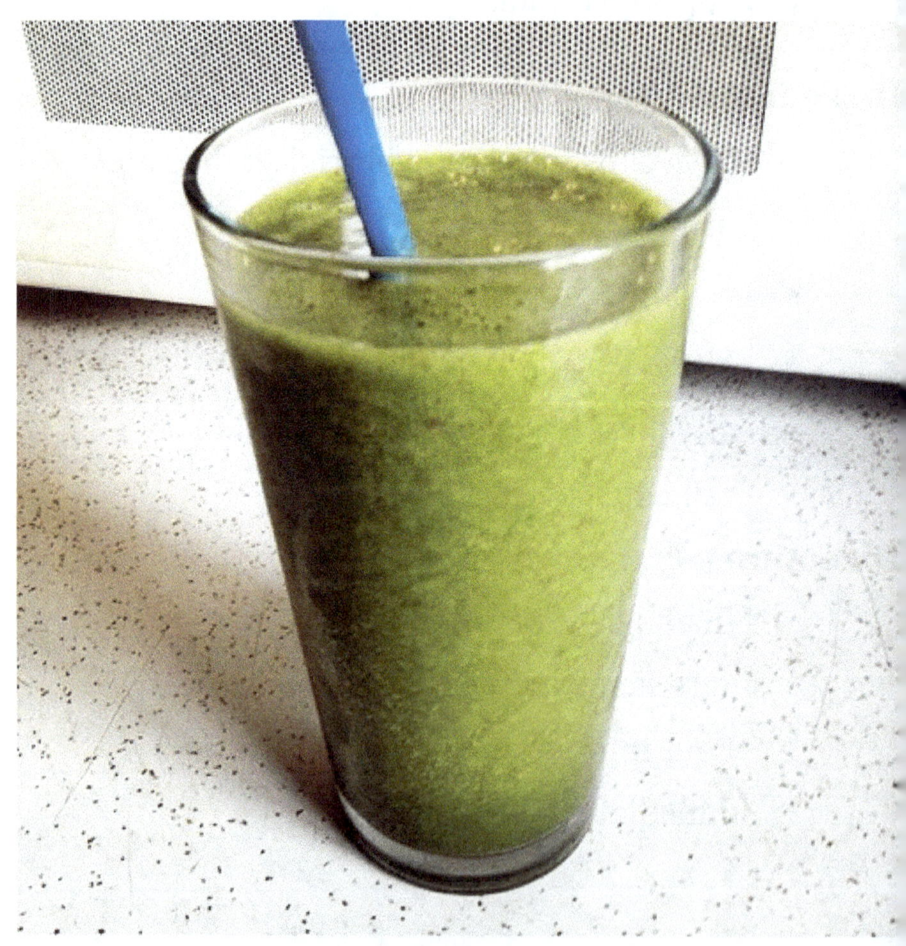

Tomato And Zucchini Sauté

Servings: 6

Cooking Time: 43 Minutes

Ingredients:

- Vegetable oil – 1 tablespoon
- Tomatoes (chopped) – 2
- Green bell pepper (chopped) – 1
- Black pepper (freshly ground) – as per taste
- Onion (sliced) – 1
- Zucchini (peeled) – 2 pounds and cut into 1-inch-thick slices
- Salt – as per taste
- Uncooked white rice – ¼ cup

Directions:

1. Begin by getting a nonstick pan and putting it over low heat. Stream in the oil and allow it to heat through.

2. Put in the onions and sauté for about 3 minutes.

3. Then pour in the zucchini and green peppers. Mix well and spice with black pepper and salt.

4. Reduce the heat and cover the pan with a lid. Allow the veggies cook on low for 5 minutes.

5. While you're done, put in the water and rice. Place the lid back on and cook on low for 20 minutes.

Nutrition Info: Calories: 94 calories per serving; Fat – 2.8 g; Protein – 3.2 g; Carbs – 16.1 g

Banana Matcha Breakfast Smoothie

Servings: 1

Cooking Time: None

Ingredients:

- 1 cup fat-free milk
- 1 medium banana, sliced
- ¼ cup frozen chopped pineapple
- ½ cup ice cubes
- 1 tablespoon matcha powder
- ¼ teaspoon ground cinnamon
- Liquid stevia extract, to taste

Directions:

1. Combine the ingredients in a blender.
2. Pulse the mixture several times to chop the ingredients.
3. Blend for 30 to 60 seconds until smooth and well combined.

4. Sweeten to taste with liquid stevia extract, if desired.

5. Pour into a glass and serve immediately.

Nutrition Info: Calories 230, Total Fat 0.4g, Saturated Fat 0.1g, Total Carbs 44.9g, Net Carbs 38g, Protein 12.6g, Sugar 30.9g, Fiber 6.9g, Sodium 135mg

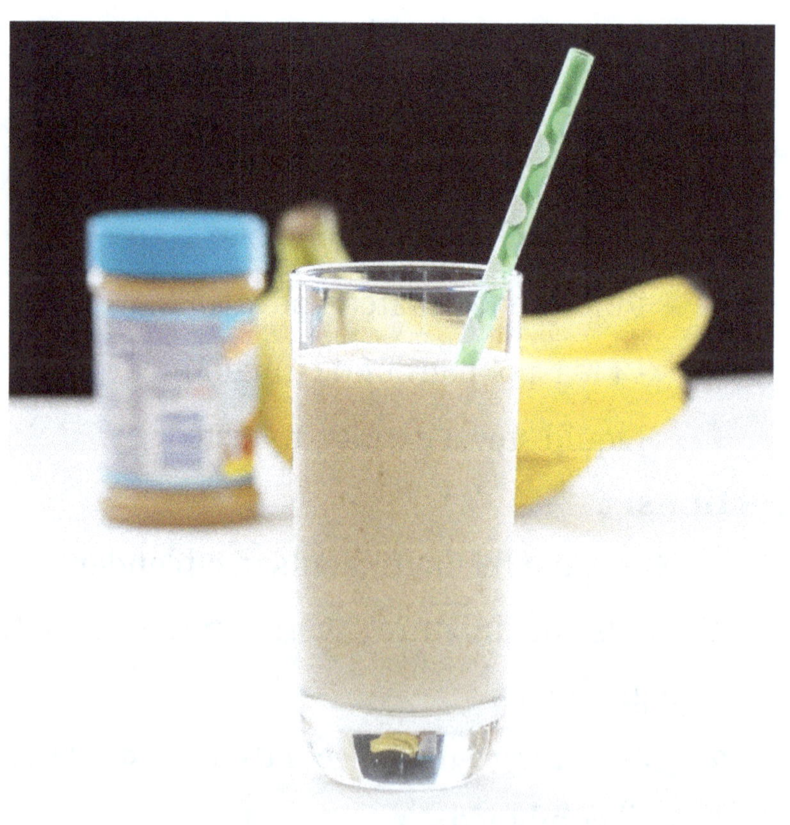

Tofu And Vegetable Scramble

Servings: 2

Cooking Time: 15 Minutes

Ingredients:

- Firm tofu (drained) – 16 ounces
- Sea salt – 1/2 teaspoon
- Garlic powder – 1 teaspoon
- Fresh coriander – for garnishing
- Red onion – 1/2 medium
- Cumin powder – 1 teaspoon
- Lemon juice – for topping
- Green bell pepper – 1 medium
- Garlic powder – 1 teaspoon
- Fresh coriander – for garnishing
- Red onion – 1/2 medium
- Cumin powder – 1 teaspoon
- Lemon juice – for topping

Directions:

1. Begin by preparing the ingredients. For this, you are to extract the seeds of the tomato and green bell pepper. Shred the onion, bell pepper, and tomato into small cubes.

2. Get a small mixing bowl and position the fairly hard tofu inside it. Make use of your hands to break the fairly hard tofu. Arrange aside.

3. Get a nonstick pan and add in the onion, tomato, and bell pepper. Mix and cook for about 3 minutes.

4. Put the somewhat hard crumbled tofu to the pan and combine well.

5. Get a small bowl and put in the water, turmeric, garlic powder, cumin powder, and chili powder. Combine well and stream it over the tofu and vegetable mixture.

6. Allow the tofu and vegetable crumble cook with seasoning for 5 minutes. Continuously stir so that the pan is not holding the ingredients.

7. Drizzle the tofu scramble with chili flakes
   and salt. Combine well.

8. Transfer the prepared scramble to a serving
   bowl and give it a proper spray of lemon juice.

9. Finalize by garnishing with pure and neat
   coriander. Serve while hot!

Nutrition Info: Calories: 238 calories per serving; Carbohydrates – 16.6 g; Fat – 11 g

Basil And Tomato Baked Eggs

Servings: 4

Cooking Time: 15 Minutes

Ingredients:

- 1 garlic clove, minced
- 1 cup canned tomatoes
- ¼ cup fresh basil leaves, roughly chopped
- 1/2 teaspoon chili powder
- 1 tablespoon olive oil
- 4 whole eggs
- Salt and pepper to taste

Directions:

1. Preheat your oven to 375 degrees F
2. Take a small baking dish and grease with olive oil
3. Add garlic, basil, tomatoes chili, olive oil into a dish and stir

4. Crackdown eggs into a dish, keeping space between the two

5. Sprinkle the whole dish with salt and pepper

6. Place in oven and cook for 12 minutes until eggs are set and tomatoes are bubbling

7. Serve with basil on top

8. Enjoy!

Nutrition Info: Calories: 235; Fat: 16g; Carbohydrates: 7g; Protein: 14g

Cream Cheese Pancakes

Servings: 1

Cooking Time: 5 Minutes

Ingredients:

- 2 oz cream cheese
- 2 eggs
- ½ tsp cinnamon
- 1 tbsp keto coconut flour
- ½ to 1 packet of Stevia

Directions:

1. Skillet with butter the pan or coconut oil on medium-high.
2. Make them as you would normal pancakes.
3. Cook and flip one side to cook the other side!
4. Top with some butter and/or sugar-free syrup.

Nutrition Info: 340 cal.30g fat 7g protein 3g carbs

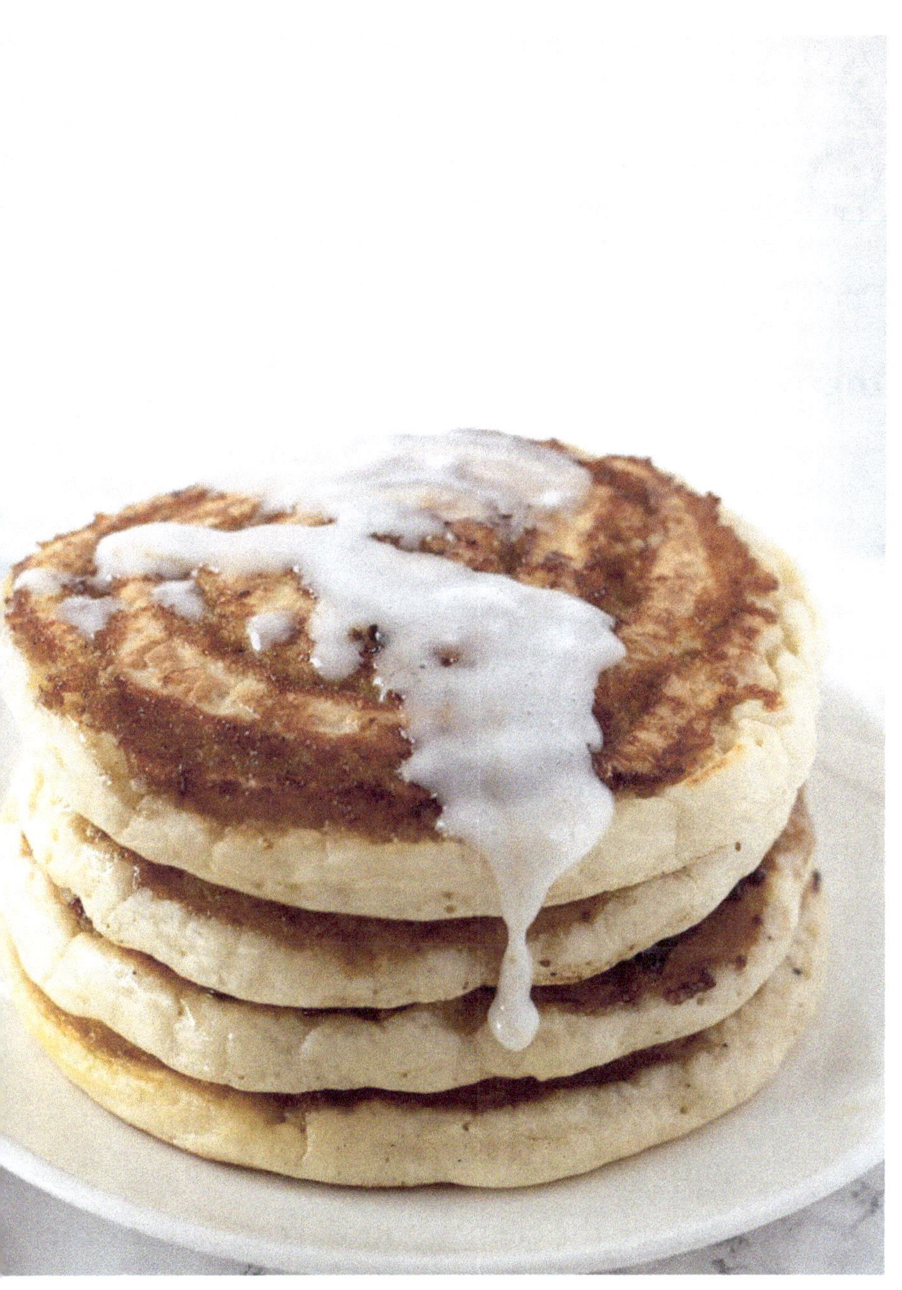

Chia And Coconut Pudding

Servings: 2

Cooking Time: 5 Minutes

Ingredients:

- Light coconut milk – 7 ounces
- Liquid stevia – 3 to 4 drops
- Kiwi – 1
- Chia seeds – ¼ cup
- Clementine – 1
- Shredded coconut (unsweetened)

Directions:

1. Begin by getting a mixing bowl and putting in the light coconut milk. Set in the liquid stevia to sweeten the milk. Combine well.
2. Put the chia seeds to the milk and whisk until well-combined. Arrange aside.
3. Scrape the clementine and carefully extract the skin from the wedges. Leave aside.

4. Also, scrape the kiwi and dice it into small pieces.

5. Get a glass vessel and gather the pudding. For this, position the fruits at the bottom of the jar; then put a dollop of chia pudding. Then spray the fruits and then put another layer of chia pudding.

6. Finalize by garnishing with the rest of the fruits and chopped coconut.

Nutrition Info: Calories: 201 calories per serving; Protein – 5.4 g; Fat – 10 g; Carbs – 22.8 g

Buckwheat Grouts Breakfast Bowl

Servings: 4

Cooking Time: 10 To 12 Minutes

Ingredients:

- 3 cups skim milk
- 1 cup buckwheat grouts
- ¼ cup chia seeds
- 2 teaspoons vanilla extract
- 1/2 teaspoon ground cinnamon
- Pinch salt
- 1 cup water
- 1/2 cup unsalted pistachios
- 2 cups sliced fresh strawberries
- ¼ cup cacao nibs (optional)

Directions:

1. In a large bowl, stir together the milk, groats, chia seeds, vanilla, cinnamon, and salt. Cover and refrigcratc overnight.

2. The next morning, transfer the soaked mixture to a medium pot and add the water. Bring to a boil over medium-high heat, reduce the heat to maintain a simmer, and cook for 10 to 12 minutes, until the buckwheat is tender and thickened.

3. Transfer to bowls and serve, topped with the pistachios, strawberries, and cacao nibs (if using).

Nutrition Info: Calories: 340; Total fat: 8g; Saturated fat: 1g; Protein: 15g; Carbs: 52g; Sugar: 14g; Fiber: 10g; Cholesterol: 4mg; Sodium: 140mg

Mashed Cauliflower

Servings: 6

Cooking Time: 10 Minutes

Ingredients:

- 1 cauliflower head
- 1/8 cup plain yogurt, skim milk or butter
- 1 red chili, diced
- 1 tomato, sliced
- ½ chopped onion
- What you will need from the store cupboard:
- 1 garlic clove, optional
- Salt and pepper
- Paprika to taste

Directions:

1. Steam the cauliflower till it becomes tender.
2. You can steam with a garlic clove as well.
3. Now cut your cauliflower into small pieces.
4. Keep in your blender with yogurt, butter or milk.
5. Season with pepper and salt. Whip until it gets smooth.
6. Pour the cauliflower into a small baking dish.
7. Sprinkle the paprika.
8. Bake in the oven till it becomes bubbly.

Nutrition Info: Calories 57, Carbohydrates 12g, Total Fat 0g, Protein 4g, Fiber 5g, Sodium 91mg, Sugars 5g

Quinoa Porridge

Servings: 2

Cooking Time: 20 Minutes

Ingredients:

- 1 cup dry quinoa, rinsed
- 1½ cups unsweetened almond milk
- 1 teaspoon vanilla extract
- 1 teaspoon ground cinnamon
- 2 tablespoons maple syrup
- 4 tablespoons peanut butter
- ¼ cup fresh strawberries, hulled and chopped
- ¼ cup fresh blueberries

Directions:

1. In a small pan, place quinoa, almond milk, vanilla extract, and cinnamon over medium heat and bring to a boil.

2. Now, adjust the heat to low and simmer, covered for about 15 minutes or until all the liquid is absorbed.

3. Remove the pan of quinoa from heat and stir in maple syrup and peanut butter.

4. Serve warm with the topping of berries.

Nutrition Info: Calories 608 Total Fat 24 g Saturated Fat 4.2 g Cholesterol 0 mg Sodium 289 mg Total Carbs 81 g Fiber 10 g Sugar 17.9 g Protein 21.1 g

Vanilla Mixed Berry Smoothie

Servings: 1

Cooking Time: None

Ingredients:

- 1 cup fat-free milk
- ½ cup nonfat Greek yogurt, plain
- ½ cup frozen blueberries
- ¼ cup frozen strawberries
- 3 to 4 ice cubes
- 1 teaspoon fresh lemon juice
- Liquid stevia extract, to taste

Directions:

1. Combine the ingredients in a blender.
2. Pulse the mixture several times to chop the ingredients.
3. Blend for 30 to 60 seconds until smooth and well combined.

4.   Sweeten to taste with liquid stevia extract, if desired.

5.   Pour into a glass and serve immediately.

Nutrition Info: Calories 220, Total Fat 0.3g, Saturated Fat 0g, Total Carbs 31.6g, Net Carbs 28.3g, Protein 21.6g, Sugar 27.3g, Fiber 3.3g, Sodium 204mg

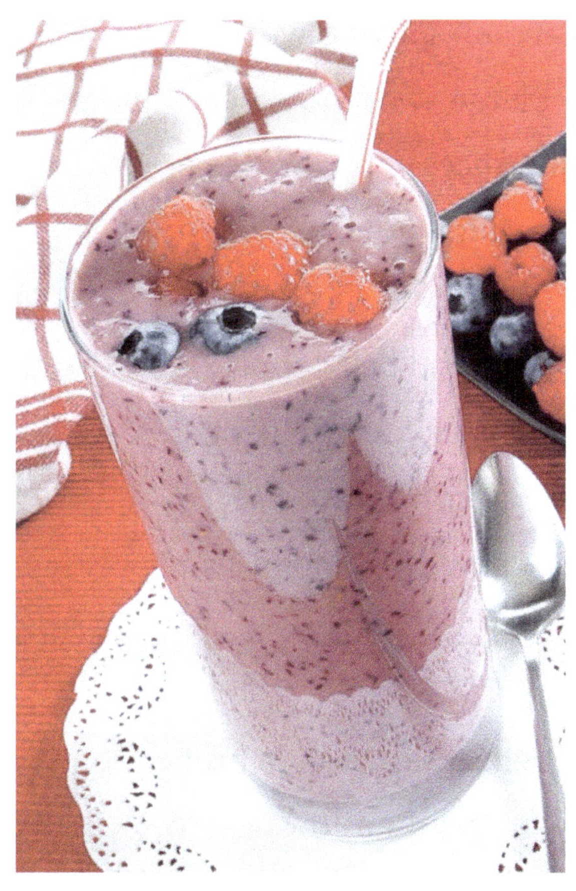

Veggie Frittata

Servings: 6

Cooking Time: 25 Minutes

Ingredients:

- 1 tablespoon olive oil
- 1 large sweet potato, cut and peeled into thin slices
- 1 yellow squash, sliced
- 1 zucchini, sliced
- ½ of red bell pepper, seeded and sliced
- ½ of yellow bell pepper, seeded and sliced
- 8 eggs
- Salt and ground black pepper, as required
- 2 tablespoons fresh cilantro, chopped finely

Directions:

1. Preheat the oven to broiler.
2. over medium-low heat, cook the sweet potato for about 6-7 minutes.

3.   Add the yellow squash, zucchini and bell peppers and cook for about 3-4 minutes.

4.   Meanwhile, in a bowl, add the eggs, salt and black pepper and beat until well combined.

5.   Pour egg mixture over vegetables mixture.

6.   Transfer the skillet in the oven and broil for about 3-4 minutes or until top becomes golden brown.

7.   With a sharp knife, cut the frittata in desired size slices and serve with the garnishing of cilantro.

Nutrition Info: Calories 143 Total Fat 8.4 g Saturated Fat 2.2 g Cholesterol 218 mg Total Carbs 9.3 g Sugar 4.2 g Fiber 1.1 g Sodium 98 mg Potassium 408 mg Protein 8.9 g

Cinnamon Rolls

Servings: 10

Cooking Time: 20 Minutes

Ingredients:

- 1 instant yeast packet
- 1 egg, large
- ¾ cups of whole milk
- 2-3/4 cups of flour
- 1 tablespoon ground cinnamon
- What you will need from the store cupboard:
- 4 tablespoons of butter, melted and unsalted
- ¾ teaspoon salt
- 2 tablespoons of maple syrup

Directions:

1. First, prepare your dough. Warm the milk and whisk in the yeast.

2. Keep it aside so that the yeast becomes foamy.

3. Beat the remaining butter, egg, flour, and salt until everything combines well.

4. Include ¼ cup flour. Knead your dough for a minute.

5. Line your cooker with parchment paper.

6. Create the filling. Create small rectangles with your dough and apply butter on top.

7. Add cinnamon. Sprinkle butter on top

8. Roll the dough up. Cut into small pieces. Cook covered.

9. Take out and then whisk in the milk and maple syrup for the icing.

10. Drizzle some milk over your rolls.

Nutrition Info: Calories 240, Carbohydrates 41g, Cholesterol 33mg, Total Fat 7g, Protein 4g, Fiber 4g, Sodium 254mg

Whole-grain Pancakes

Servings: 4 To 6

Cooking Time: 15 Minutes

Ingredients:

- 2 cups whole-wheat pastry flour
- 4 teaspoons baking powder
- 2 teaspoons ground cinnamon
- 1/2 teaspoon salt
- 2 cups skim milk, plus more as needed
- 2 large eggs
- 1 tablespoon honey
- Nonstick cooking spray
- Maple syrup, for serving
- Fresh fruit, for serving

Directions:

1. In a large bowl, stir together the flour, baking powder, cinnamon, and salt.

2. Add the milk, eggs, and honey, and stir well to combine. If needed, add more milk, 1 tablespoon at a time, until there are no dry spots and you has a pourable batter.

3. Heat a large skillet over medium-high heat, and spray it with cooking spray.

4. Using a ¼-cup measuring cup, scoop 2 or 3 pancakes into the skillet at a time. Cook for a couple of minutes, until bubbles form on the surface of the pancakes, flip, and cook for 1 to 2 minutes more, until golden brown and cooked through. Repeat with the remaining batter.

5. Serve topped with maple syrup or fresh fruit.

Nutrition Info: Calories: 392; Total fat: 4g; Saturated fat: 1g; Protein: 15g; Carbs: 71g; Sugar: 11g; Fiber: 9g; Cholesterol: 95mg; Sodium: 396mg

Granola With Fruits

Servings: 6

Cooking Time: 35 Minutes

Ingredients:

- 3 cups quick cooking oats
- 1 cup almonds, sliced
- ½ cup wheat germ
- 3 tablespoons butter
- 1 teaspoon ground cinnamon
- 1 cup honey
- 3 cups whole grain cereal flakes
- ½ cup raisins
- ½ cup dried cranberries
- ½ cup dates, pitted and chopped

Directions:

1. Preheat your oven to 325 degrees F.
2. Place the almonds on a baking sheet.
3. Bake for 15 minutes.

4. Mix the wheat germ, butter, cinnamon and honey in a bowl.

5. Add the toasted almonds and oats.

6. Mix well.

7. Spread on the baking sheet.

8. Bake for 20 minutes.

9. Mix with the rest of the ingredients.

10. Let cool and serve.

Nutrition Info: Calories 210 Total Fat 7 g Saturated Fat 2 g Cholesterol 5 mg Sodium 58 mg Total Carbohydrate 36 g Dietary Fiber 4 g Total Sugars 2 g Protein 5 g Potassium 250 mg

Egg Muffins

Servings: 6

Cooking Time: 20 Minutes

Ingredients:

- 1 tbsp green pesto
- 3 oz/75g shredded cheese
- 5 oz/150g cooked bacon
- 1 scallion, chopped
- 6 eggs

Directions:

1. You should set your oven to 350°F/175°C.
2. Place liners in a regular cupcake tin. This will help with easy removal and storage.
3. Beat the eggs with pepper, salt, and the pesto. Mix in the cheese.
4. Pour the eggs into the cupcake tin and top with the bacon and scallion.
5. Cook for 15-20 minutes

Nutrition Info: 190 cal.15g fat 7g protein 4g carbs.

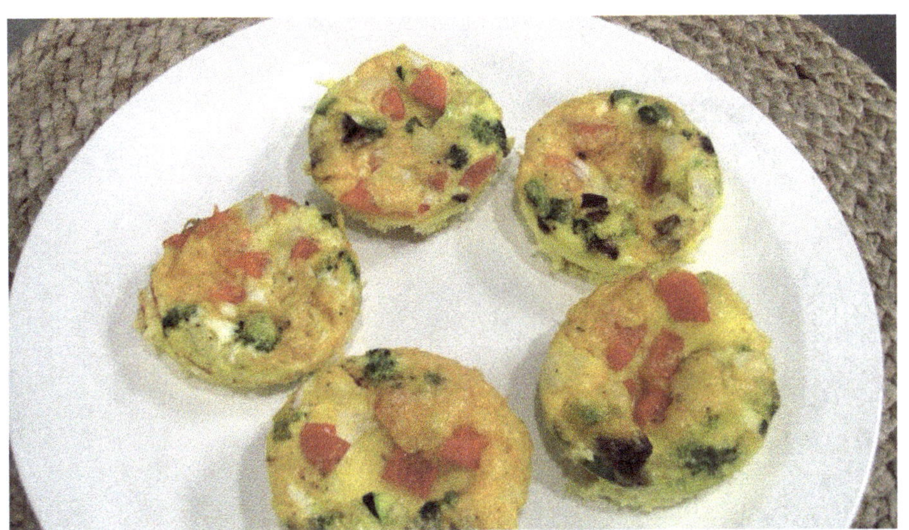

Eggs On The Go

Servings: 4

Cooking Time: 5 Minutes

Ingredients:

- 4 oz/110g bacon, cooked
- Pepper
- Salt
- 12 eggs

Directions:

1. You should set your oven to 200°C.
2. Place liners in a regular cupcake tin. This will help with easy removal and storage.
3. Crack an egg into each of the cups and sprinkle some bacon onto each of them. Season with some pepper and salt.
4. Bake for 15 minutes, or until the eggs are set.

Nutrition Info: 75 cal. 6g fat 8g protein 1g carbs.

Breakfast Mix

Servings: 1

Cooking Time: 5 Minutes

Ingredients:

- 5 tbsp coconut flakes, unsweetened
- 7 tbsp hemp seeds
- 5 tbsp flaxseed, ground
- 2 tbsp sesame, ground
- 2 tbsp cocoa, dark, unsweetened

Directions:

1. Grind the sesame and flaxseed.
2. only grind the sesame seeds for a small period..
3. Mix all ingredients in a jar and shake it well.
4. Keep refrigerated until ready to eat.

5. Serve softened with black coffee or even with still water and add coconut oil if you want to increase the fat content. It also blends well with cream or with mascarpone cheese.

Nutrition Info: 150 cal.9g fat 8g protein 4g carbs.

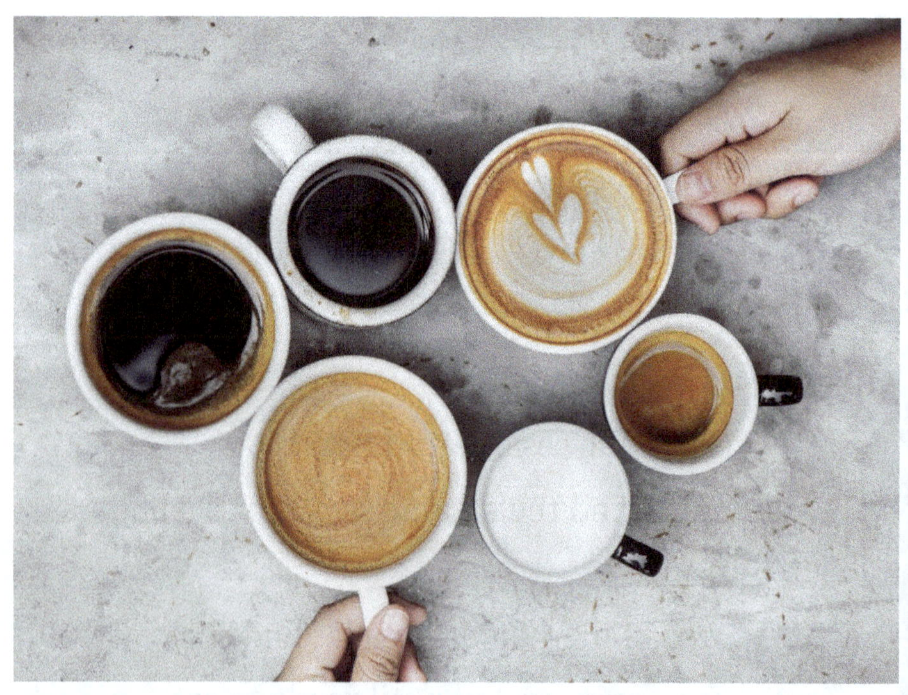

Lovely Porridge

Servings: 2

Cooking Time: Nil

Ingredients:

- 2 tablespoons coconut flour
- 2 tablespoons vanilla protein powder
- 3 tablespoons Golden Flaxseed meal
- 1 and 1/2 cups almond milk, unsweetened
- Powdered erythritol

Directions:

1. Take a bowl and mix in flaxseed meal, protein powder, coconut flour and mix well
2. Add mix to the saucepan (placed over medium heat)
3. Add almond milk and stir, let the mixture thicken

4. Add your desired amount of sweetener and serve

5. Enjoy!

Nutrition Info: Calories: 259; Fat: 13g; Carbohydrates: 5g; Protein: 16g

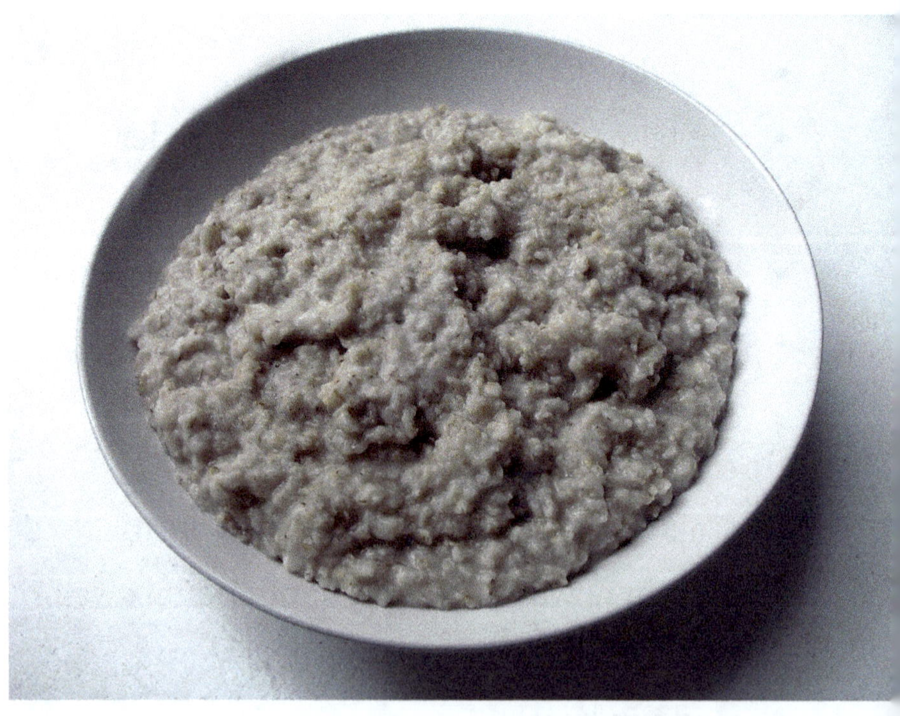

Vegetable Omelet

Servings: 4

Cooking Time: 25 Minutes

Ingredients:

- ½ cup yellow summer squash, chopped
- ½ cup canned diced tomatoes with herbs, drained
- ½ ripe avocado, pitted and chopped
- ½ cup cucumber, chopped
- 2 eggs
- 2 tablespoons water
- Salt and pepper to taste
- 1 teaspoon dried basil, crushed
- Cooking spray
- ¼ cup low-fat Monterey Jack cheese, shredded
- Chives, chopped

Directions:

1. In a bowl, mix the squash, tomatoes, avocado and cucumber.

2. In another bowl, mix the eggs, water, salt, pepper and basil.

3. Spray oil on a pan over medium heat.

4. Pour egg mixture on the pan.

5. Put the vegetable mixture on top of the egg.

6. Lift and fold.

7. Cook until the egg has set.

8. Sprinkle cheese and chives on top.

Nutrition Info: Calories 128 Total Fat 6 g Saturated Fat 2 g Cholesterol 97 mg Sodium 357 mg Total Carbohydrate 7 g Dietary Fiber 3 g Total Sugars 4 g Protein 12 g Potassium 341 mg